Exercise and the Coronary Patient

Exercise
and the
Coronary
Patient

E. R. NYE, M.B., PH.D., F.R.A.C.P.
and
P. GAY WOOD, N.Z.R.P., N.Z.T.P.

WOLFE PUBLISHING LIMITED
10 Earlham Street London WC2

First published in New Zealand in 1971
by Whitcombe & Tombs Ltd
P.O. Box 7495, Christchurch, New Zealand
and in the United Kingdom in 1971
by Wolfe Publishing Ltd
10 Earlham Street, London W.C.2

PRINTED IN GREAT BRITAIN
BY EBENEZER BAYLIS AND SON LTD
THE TRINITY PRESS, WORCESTER, AND LONDON

Preface

THE PURPOSE of this book is to give a simple account of the exercise programme that we have devised for patients who have recovered from a heart attack.

Sections on anatomical, physiological, pathological, clinical and epidemiological aspects relevant to the subject matter are designed to help physiotherapists and physical educationists obtain a broad view of the field without having to refer to specialist literature.

Medical practitioners will probably wish to refer mainly to the sections dealing directly with the exercise programme.

This work is not intended as a 'do-it-yourself' manual for patients and it is stressed that while the running of an exercise programme for coronary patients is not unduly difficult it does entail a regular time commitment by an interested physician and an assistant.

Finally, it is hoped that an interest in the therapeutic aspects of physical activity may lead to a greater appreciation of the preventive value of exercise.

In the Appendix is reproduced the WHO protocol for exercise testing of population groups prepared under the direction of Professor K. Lange Andersen of Oslo. This protocol sets out in detail the measures necessary for assessment of physical fitness and is essentially an implication of the screening procedure and precautions described in the main part of the text. The protocol is reproduced through the courtesy of Professor Andersen and the World Health Organisation.

NOTE: Reference numbers are included in the text to sources listed in the Bibliography (page 75).

Contents

		page
Introduction		9
Chapter		
1	Anatomy and Physiology of the Coronary Circulation	13
2	Pathology and Clinical Aspects of Coronary Heart Disease	17
3	Effect of Exercise—General	25
4	Effect of Exercise on the Cardiovascular System	31
5	Considerations in Planning an Exercise Programme	35
6	The Formal Exercise Programme	41
7	Epidemiological Considerations	61
8	The Coronary Club	65
9	The Physical and Psychological Effects of the Exercise Programme on Coronary Patients	69
Bibliography		75
Appendix		79

Introduction

THE CONCEPT of the therapeutic value of 'rest' has been a corner-stone of medicine and surgery for so many hundreds of years that it is not surprising that little thought has been given to the possibility that in some areas of treatment too much rest might be undesirable. It is well known that enforced immobilisation may lead to muscle wasting and osteoporosis, but as long as the consequences of inadequate immobilisation present more serious difficulties, such as an unstable fracture, the presence of remediable muscle weakness is a price worth paying.

The human body is, however, built for action. It can be trained to run at twenty miles an hour for short distances, run at least twenty-six miles non-stop, climb mountains 29,000 feet high and, with a bit of assistance, walk on the moon. In all these activities the heart plays a key role by supplying the working muscles with blood. In the treatment of the commonest mortal disease in the community, coronary heart disease, physical rest of the patient, and therefore of the heart, is the main measure used in dealing with the early phases of the illness. There

9

are good grounds for enforced rest at this stage. However, the damaged heart has usually healed by six weeks. For generations physicians have mostly enjoined their coronary patient to 'take things quietly' once they have recovered from a coronary attack. In the last ten years, though, an increasing number of doctors have begun to wonder if the indefinite protraction of relative physical inactivity is either desirable or necessary. There is currently a more liberal attitude on the part of many physicians, who encourage their patients to get up earlier after a heart-attack and to lead a more active existence after recovery where possible. The abandonment of the more conservative attitude to physical activity may probably be carried too far and at present there is no study which compares accurately the progress of patients treated conservatively, either early or late in the illness, with similar patients treated on more aggressive lines.

Many physicians who have grown familiar with the use of physical exercise as a recuperative measure after patients have survived three months from the original attack have, however, become enthusiastic over this form of treatment. In studies carried out in Canada, the United States, Scandinavia and Israel there is no clear evidence that properly selected patients come to harm from physical activity programmes; in fact, they appear to derive both symptomatic and psychological benefits. In spite of the optimism over the physical programmes, there is nonetheless no mandate at present for the general recommendation of this form of treatment in all patients, and all published work in the field emphasises the need to assess patients carefully both before and during the exercise programmes. It is indeed possible that part of the success of these programmes depends on the confidence that patients receive from knowing that they are under the supervision of trained medical personnel.

The successful application of an exercise programme for convalescent coronary patients in the New Zealand setting has encouraged us to prepare this manual as a guide to others interested in this particular area of rehabilitation.

It is appreciated that some aspects of rehabilitation have been neglected in this book. Thus it has not been thought necessary to dwell at length on the very important question of giving the patient an accurate but simple account of the nature of his disorder. Again, the question of resettlement of a patient into employment has not been dealt with, although this question does arise in our work.

Finally, rehabilitation in the present context means rehabilitation, not necessarily only for the working patient, but also very often as an important measure allowing the retired patient to enjoy a fuller life.

CHAPTER 1

Anatomy and Physiology of the Coronary Circulation

A BETTER APPRECIATION of the postulated role of exercise in the treatment of patients with coronary heart disease can be obtained by some understanding of the normal anatomy and physiology of the coronary circulation.

ANATOMY

Blood is supplied to the heart muscle by the left and right coronary arteries, arising respectively from the left and anterior aortic sinuses. Both arteries wind round the atrio-ventricular groove and the left artery gives off a large anterior interventricular branch near its origin. While the left coronary artery supplies mainly the left ventricle and the right artery supplies the right ventricle, there is considerable individual variability in the perfusion area of the two arteries. Little or no functional anastomosis occurs between the two arteries. Penetrating branches of the arteries supply blood to the heart muscle, except for the endocardium which is in direct contact with the blood inside the heart chambers.

The wall of a coronary artery is structurally similar to other arteries and consists of an inner, smooth endothelial lining, an internal elastic layer, a muscular middle coat (media) and an outer adventitial layer of connective tissue. The medial and adventitial coats of the arteries receive blood carried by vasa vasora.

The venous return from the heart is carried by cardiac veins which open into the right atrium via the coronary sinus and anterior coronary veins.

PHYSIOLOGY

The supply of blood to the heart via the coronary arteries fluctuates, since the intramural branches of the arteries are subject to the pressure generated by the heart muscle with each contraction. It can indeed be shown that coronary flow falls in part of the left ventricular muscle during ventricular systole and may be zero in the sub-endocardial region. As a consequence much of the coronary flow depends on the diastolic pressure in the aorta produced by the elastic recoil of the aorta coupled with the peripheral systemic resistance. It is clear, therefore, that the shorter the diastolic interval, as during periods of rapid heart rate, the shorter the time available for coronary perfusion. Also if the forward flow produced by the heart is deficient by reason of inefficient action, such as might be produced by disordered rhythm, coronary perfusion may be less than optimal. The relation between ventricular pressure, aortic pressure and coronary flow is shown diagrammatically in Figure 1.

The coronary arteries not only provide the blood supply to contracting cardiac muscle but also to the conducting system of the heart. Blood is usually supplied

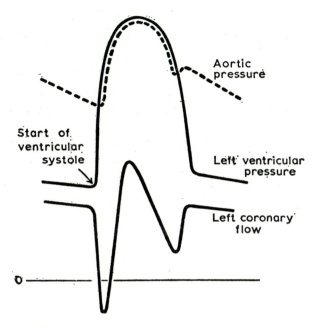

Aortic
pressure

Start of
ventricular
systole

Left ventricular
pressure

Left coronary
flow

o

FIG. I   *Pressure changes in the left ventricle and aorta related to flow in the left coronary artery during one cardiac cycle.*

to the part of the interventricular septum containing the atrio-ventricular node by an arterial branch (the nodal artery) arising from the right coronary artery; less commonly by a branch of the left coronary artery. Thus an interruption of the blood supply to the atrio-ventricular node, or other parts of the conducting system, can cause complete or partial conduction block. This leads in some cases to an abnormally slow fixed heart rate which may be incompatible with adequate cerebral and coronary perfusion. Sudden stoppage of blood flow to the nodal artery may also lead to cardiac arrest.

VARIATION IN CORONARY BLOOD FLOW

While aortic pressure is the main determinant of coronary flow, experimental studies indicate that control mechanisms involving dilation or constriction of the coronary arteries also exist. Thus exercise-induced tachycardia can increase coronary flow in normal subjects in spite of the decreased diastolic period available for perfusion.

Experimental studies in animals also indicate that a fall in blood volume produced by blood loss may also give rise to coronary vasodilation, a mechanism which would tend to protect the heart muscle from ischaemic damage.

CHAPTER 2

Pathology and Clinical Aspects of Coronary Heart Disease

PATHOLOGY

By far the commonest cause of coronary heart disease is narrowing of the coronary arteries by the process of atheroma formation. The term 'atherosclerosis' is widely used to describe the fully developed disease process.

Atherosclerosis is a form of arterial disease which is widespread in vertebrate animals and much study on the factors which promote and retard the process has been carried out, chiefly in such animals as birds, rabbits and dogs. As a result of the experimental studies, and observations on human pathology, four main stages are described, of which the first is not universally regarded as necessarily the forerunner of the remainder. These stages (shown in Figure 2) are:

(1) THE FATTY-STREAK. This is seen as accumulations of fatty material in foam cells, below the intima of the artery but not invading the media. The fatty material consists of triglycerides, cholesterol esters, cholesterol

and some phospholipids. This fatty streak can be demonstrated by the use of special stains in the arterial walls of infants and it has been disputed whether or not the fatty streak is the forerunner of the later stages. There seems no doubt that these lesions are potentially reversible.

(2) THE ATHEROMATOUS PLAQUE. This consists of a patch of lipid material in the sub-intimal region, some of the material lying free and not confined to foam cells. Plaques are usually easily seen through the intima of the opened artery and the lipid material and associated debris has a porridgy consistency. Some thickening of the sub-intimal region is now obvious on sectioning the artery, with encroachment of the disease process on the muscle coat of the arterial media. It seems likely that this stage is potentially reversible.

(3) THE FIBRO-FATTY PLAQUE. This is similar to the foregoing but there is now a fibrotic reaction in the plaque as a result of invasion of fibroblasts. The arterial media is invaded and the resulting deformation of the arterial wall leads to altered physical and physiological properties of the artery. The lesion is probably only partly reversible.

(4) THE FIBROUS PLAQUE. The dominant material is now fibrous tissue and on the inner lining of the cut artery is seen a raised flattened area of rigid collagen. There is considerable deformation of the arterial wall and its physical properties are greatly changed. Calcification may be present. The lesion is unlikely to be reversible.

While lesions (3) and (4) are separately described, they often exist in various degrees of transition and patches of diseased artery may be separated by areas of apparently normal tissue.

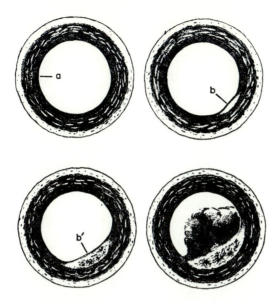

FIG. 2 *Diagrammatic cross section of coronary artery showing progression of atheroma lesion. Normal intima* (a), *early plaque* (b) *and later stage in plaque formation* (b¹). *The fourth figure shows the presence of a thrombus on a plaque.*

The distribution of the atheromatous lesions appears to be not entirely a random event but possibly influenced by certain physical and perhaps structural factors. It has been noticed that the plaques are more prominent at arterial bifurcations and also that some parts of the arterial tree are more prone to the disease changes than others.

CORONARY ATHEROSCLEROSIS

The presence of the atheromatous lesions in the coronary arteries and their main branches leads to narrowing which, in turn, reduces the flow of blood to the heart muscle. It should be noted that since flow through a tube is proportional, among other things, to the cross-sectional area of the tube, a reduction of the cross-sectional area produces a reduction in flow which is inversely proportional to the square of the radius. Thus halving of the radius of an artery produces a reduction in flow, other things being equal, to one-quarter of the original value. It is also probable that irregularities produced by the patchy lesion of atheroma lead to turbulent flow in the affected vessels, which could lead to less efficient perfusion.

The narrowed coronary arteries may also become suddenly and completely occluded by the formation of a thrombus, which, in clinical terms, leads to a 'heart-attack' or myocardial infarction. It should be noted, however, that the clinical and pathological event of myocardial infarction, which means death of the heart muscle served by the affected artery, cannot always be demonstrated to be due to blockage of the artery by a thrombus at post-mortem examination. This puzzling fact still requires explanation.

CLINICAL CORONARY HEART DISEASE

The clinical manifestations of coronary heart disease may be categorised as follows:

1. *Angina pectoris*

Firstly, chest pain which occurs when heart muscle becomes ischaemic. This pain may occur when the patient, either as a result of exercise or emotion, causes the heart to work harder. A point is reached when the narrowed coronary arteries cannot meet the heart's increased need for blood and the patient experiences a sense of discomfort in the centre of the chest which is variously described as gripping, band like, or a sense of constriction or heaviness. The pain may radiate to the inside of the arms, usually the left, and to neck and jaw. The pain passes off when the patient rests, or uses a drug such as glyceryl trinitrate.

The amount of effort required to bring on the pain is variable, even for the same patient, who may find only certain activities will bring on the pain while other, and apparently more severe, activities may fail to do so.

2. *Myocardial Infarction*

The pain of myocardial infarction, which occurs usually when an irreversible stoppage of blood to part of the heart muscle has taken place, is similar to that of angina pectoris but often more severe and is not relieved by rest or by glyceryl trinitrate. The patient may also feel faint, nauseated and anxious. If the heart's action as a pump is impaired by the damage to the muscle, the patient may experience shortness of breath.

3. *Heart Failure*

A heart severely damaged by ischaemic disease, either as the result of an acute or insidious process, may fail to operate efficiently when the patient exerts himself. As the left ventricle is most commonly involved by ischaemic disease, the symptoms of left ventricular failure, shortness of breath on effort, may trouble the patient. In mild cases the symptoms may only occur on moderate activity. In more severe cases very slight activity, such as dressing or even talking may provoke this distressing symptom. The condition of left ventricular failure in its more severe form is often accompanied by shortness of breath at night and the patient finds he has to sit propped up to sleep.

The symptom of shortness of breath is due mainly to congestion of the pulmonary veins, leading to oedema and reduced lung elasticity as the left ventricle fails to put out blood passing through the pulmonary vasculature under the action of the right ventricle.

In more severe cases right ventricular failure may ensue and the patient then complains of weakness, ankle swelling, abdominal discomfort, loss of appetite. The right ventricle fails to put out blood returning to it from the venous side. The blood volume increases; the liver increases in size as a result of the high venous pressure. Oedema fluid accumulates in the extremities and fluid may accumulate in the abdominal cavity (ascites). In untreated cases the patient dies eventually of hepatic and renal failure.

4. *Palpitation*

Irregularities of the heart action may be noticed by the patient. In the patient who has ischaemic heart disease irregularities of rhythm may occur, consisting of the occasional extra beat, or runs of rapid beats, either regular or irregular in rhythm. These abnormal rhythms are particularly important clinically in the patient who has just suffered a myocardial infarction and appear to arise from abnormal excitatory foci in heart muscle bordering the infarcted area. The abnormal rhythm in the acute attack may be incompatible with the heart's action as a pump and cause death within a few minutes. The fatal rhythm that threatens the patient in the first few minutes and hours after a coronary occlusion is ventricular fibrillation. A rapid ventricular rate, such as a ventricular tachycardia, may, without being fatal of itself, so reduce the heart's efficiency that left ventricular failure may occur. Abnormally slow rhythm may also occur, such as sinus bradycardia, and heart block of varying degree. Sudden complete stoppage of the heart's action (asystole) may also occur.

5. *Shock*

The victim of a myocardial infarction may present with a shock-like state characterised by a cold, pale, clammy skin, rapid or sometimes slow, thin pulse and low blood pressure. Transient degrees of shock are not uncommon but persistence of the shock-like state for more than a short period is associated with a very poor outlook.

CHAPTER 3

Effect of Exercise — General

IT IS COMMONLY ACCEPTED that regular physical activity
brings 'physical fitness'. The definition of physical fitness
is difficult but it is fairly generally agreed that a satisfactory definition is that physical fitness is associated with
a rapid return to normal of cardiovascular and metabolic
functions after the subject stops a spell of exercise and
rests. Implicit in the definition, therefore, is the concept
of 'physical unfitness'.

The effects of exercise on the cardiovascular system
will be dealt with more fully in the next section.

EXERCISE AND THE RESPIRATORY SYSTEM

Two main sources of energy are available for muscular
activity: carbohydrate, in the form of muscle glycogen,
or glucose in the blood; fat, in the form of triglyceride in
the muscle and fatty acids, free or esterified, in the blood.
Since oxygen is required for the oxidation of the above
substances, thereby providing the chemical energy necessary for muscular contraction to occur, any increase in

25

muscular activity calls for increased oxygen transport from air to muscle. The heart is stimulated to increased activity and the transport of oxygenated blood from lungs to working muscle is hastened. The exercise is accompanied by an increase in the rate and depth of respiration which has several results. Aeration of all parts of the lung proceeds more efficiently and is accompanied by an increase in the perfusion of blood to those parts of the lungs that were less well aerated in the resting state. As a result of these changes there is a greater capacity for oxygen transfer to blood coming from the right side of the heart. Equally important is the increased capacity for the removal of carbon dioxide from the blood, now produced in increased quantity by the muscular activity.

A third, but minor, contribution made by the lungs is the increase in heat loss resulting from the transfer of heat from the body to the expired air, and the heat lost in the form of latent heat of vaporisation of the water in the alveoli and lost with the water vapour in the expired air.

The lungs are therefore playing their part, not only by providing the extra oxygen necessary for the muscular work, but also by preventing the build-up of excess carbonic acid in the blood. The functional capacity of the lungs can be gauged from the approximate figures for a male of average build:

    Minute volume at rest :   8-10 litres
       (air breathed in and out)
    Oxygen removed from
       air in 1 minute   :   300-400 millilitres
    Minute volume under conditions
       of severe exercise   :   c. 120 litres
    Oxygen removed from
       air in 1 minute   :   c. 3500 millilitres

SKELETAL MUSCLE

The immediate effect of a burst of exercise on skeletal muscle is to increase the muscle blood flow—a reasonable and readily understood response. This increase in metabolic activity is accompanied by local warming, a phenomenon which appears to increase the efficiency and speed of muscular contraction, a factor known empirically to athletes who do 'warm-up' exercises before a big event. Depending on the severity of the exercise, there may be a reduction of the glycogen content of the muscle which can be used as an energy source by the process of anaerobic glycolysis under conditions of severe exercise for brief periods. The glycogen store is replenished under conditions of rest by being built up from the blood glucose.

Regular exercise produces an increase in the fibre size of the affected muscles, which is seen as an increase in muscle bulk in the trained person. With training in certain sports, constant practice produces, as the result of facilitation of nervous pathways in the brain, the possibility of carrying out certain movements very efficiently and accurately, so that the effects of a training session on muscle bulk and strength may be less in the skilled than the unskilled. This paradoxical situation is readily understood when one sees an experienced player at, say, squash rackets or table tennis dealing skilfully and with minimum of effort with an unskilled opponent. The situation is of course different when two players of similar experience are pitted against each other.

By the same token, a manual worker who has become skilled in the performance of his work may be able to carry out his physical tasks more efficiently and more economically than the untrained person. This may explain the paradoxical clinical finding that some patients experience little or no angina when apparently active at work, but find that such a task as hedge-cutting, which is done infrequently, brings on their pain.

METABOLIC EFFECTS OF EXERCISE

As indicated earlier, muscular action depends on the transformation of chemical energy into kinetic energy. The energy source for this process is either glucose, glycogen, fatty acids or more complex lipid substances.

In the supply of energy for sudden bursts of activity, such as a spring from resting conditions, circulatory and respiratory mechanisms do not come into play soon enough to allow an adequate supply of energy from the oxidative metabolism of respiratory substrate. Under these conditions energy is released by a process of anaerobic glycolysis which leads to the production of lactic acid from glycogen. The measurement of lactic acid in the blood may be used as an index of the anaerobic sources of energy in experimental studies.

When oxygen is available, the conversion of lactic acid to pyruvic acid and thence to carbon-dioxide and water is possible.

In addition to the above, oxidative processes occur which result in the complete transformation of glycogen and lipid substances into carbon-dioxide and water.

Essentially all exercise involves both aerobic and anaerobic metabolic steps, although the balance in either direction will depend on a number of factors such as the severity of the exercise and the degree of physical fitness of the subject.

A spell of exercise which is protracted for more than a few minutes results in the release of fatty acids from the triglycerides of adipose tissue. Thus careful studies of the blood fatty acids and glycerol both during and after exercise show that there are changes consistent with the mobilisation of fat, probably through the action of such substances as noradrenaline, adrenaline and adrenal cortical hormones.

Other effects of physical activity of more than moderate degree include a reduction in the level of certain lipo-proteins, leading to reduction chiefly in the plasma triglyceride, and a rise in haemoglobin concentration due to movement of water from the vascular compartment into the interstitial compartment.

CHAPTER 4

Effect of Exercise on the Cardiovascular System

FOR CONVENIENCE OF DISCUSSION this section may be sub-divided on the basis of the acute and long-term effects of physical training on the cardiovascular system.

ACUTE EFFECT OF EXERCISE ON THE CARDIOVASCULAR SYSTEM

As indicated in the previous section, the effect of exercise is to increase the need for blood in active muscle. Vascular beds in contracting muscle are perfused both by a larger amount of blood and by a larger fraction of the cardiac output than in the resting state. In the adjustments that occur the fraction of the cardiac output to the abdominal viscera, including the kidneys, is reduced. Blood flow to the skin is also reduced, except when the need for heat loss assumes overriding import-ance and the skin vessels dilate. Blood flow to the heart increases.

31

The most obvious result of physical activity on the heart is an increase in the heart rate. The reasons for the increase in rate are not fully understood but it seems clear that at least two main factors are responsible. The first is mediated via nervous control of the heart's action and is, at least partly, under the control of higher nervous centres, since rises in heart rate *precede* exercise and changes in heart rate can be induced by emotional factors. In addition it is known that alteration in vagal tone (parasympathetic) to the sinoatrial node affects heart rate. Thus increase in vagal tone slows the heart, whereas a decrease in vagal tone produces a quickening of the heart rate. In addition, the accelerator nerve to the heart (sympathetic) causes an increase in heart rate. The control of both the parasympathetic and sympathetic nervous outflows to the heart is found in special centres in the brain stem.

However, the heart deprived of its nervous connections will also increase in rate in response to exercise, although the control mechanism appears less finely tuned.

The non-nervous control of heart rate resides chiefly in the adrenal medulla, since under the influence of emotion and exercise there is a rise in the production of the substance adrenaline (epinephrine) by the adrenal medulla. Adrenaline causes a rise in heart rate, a dilation of blood vessels in muscle, a rise in blood sugar and a sense of increased mental alertness—all effects appropriate to bodily exercise.

The effect of physical activity on the heart is not, of course, confined to change in the heart rate. The amount of blood pumped by the heart in a given time is increased; this is achieved not only by increasing the number of contractions in unit time but also by increasing the stroke volume, and it appears that this is achieved by more efficient emptying of the heart with ventricular systole.

LONG-TERM EFFECTS OF EXERCISE ON THE CARDIOVASCULAR SYSTEM

The effects of regular physical activity on the heart in normal people have been well studied and can be summarised briefly as follows, where the changes before and after training are compared:

1. There is a slowing of the resting heart rate, due to increased vagal tone.
2. There is an increase in end-diastolic volume, due to the increased time available for ventricular filling.
3. There is an increased stroke volume, which follows from 1 and 2.
4. The heart rate during exercise for a given exercise load is decreased.
5. The recovery time of the heart rate to the resting level, again after a given work quotient, is reduced.

In general terms the changes may be summarised by saying that the heart performs more efficiently by doing the same amount of work at a lower rate of contraction. The increased efficiency of the heart as the result of training is probably due, in part, to hypertrophy of the heart muscle, since in animal studies it has been shown that endurance activities for prolonged periods produces an increase in heart weight. There seems no doubt that the physiological capacity of the heart is improved by endurance training, and the capacity of the human heart to support marathon runners, four-minute milers and other great physical feats is well known.

EFFECTS OF EXERCISE ON THE CORONARY ARTERIES

Since the actively contracting heart muscle, both under conditions of rest and exercise, requires perfusion by blood, the carrying capacity of the coronary arteries may impose a limit on the amount of work that the heart can do, as occurs in the patient who suffers from angina of effort. It would, therefore, be of considerable interest, and importance, to learn if physical activity in any way influenced the size of the main coronary arteries, or the size of the alternative channels available for perfusion of the myocardium. It is worth noting, therefore, that the coronary arteries of a veteran marathon runner have been found to be two to three times larger than normal.[1] There is also some evidence from experiments with animals that exercise improves the coronary circulation, by promoting development of collateral vessels where an artificial obstruction to a main coronary branch has been made.[2]

Direct evidence of beneficial effect of long-term exercise on the coronary circulation is likely to be difficult to obtain for a number of years, or at least until safe and reliable methods are available for examining the coronary arteries. However, the available evidence, meagre though it is, would seem to suggest that beneficial effects might occur.

CHAPTER 5

Considerations in Planning an Exercise Programme

IT IS PROBABLE, but not certain, that the successful running of an exercise programme for coronary patients depends on interested and optimistic attitudes of the physician and physiotherapist themselves, as in other areas of therapy. It may be helpful also if the medical attendants are known to make some special effort to maintain an increased level of physical fitness. In the Dunedin programme the physicians in charge have made a practice of taking part in many of the patients' twice-weekly evening activities. This not only provides the supervision necessary but also encourages the patients and has been very helpful in giving the medical team considerable insight into the physical capacity of their patients. The sight of a middle-aged patient known to have sustained a full-thickness anterior infarct playing an energetic game of badminton with a student half his age is calculated to leave a lasting impression.

Regular opportunity for consultation between physician and physiotherapist has also been found invaluable. We have arranged for all follow-up appointments for patients in the programme to take place at a special clinic when both the physician and physiotherapist can discuss the progress and problems of patients. The same clinic assesses new patients and it is helpful if both members of the team can see the patient jointly at the initial interview.

SELECTION OF PATIENTS

At the initial interview and examinations the suitability of the patient for the programme has to be decided. We do not regard patients as suitable who:

1. Have symptoms of left ventricular failure, that is, shortness of breath on effort or nocturnal dyspnoea. We have been reluctant to include patients with therapeutically controlled left ventricular failure, although we do review such patients and include them in the programme if it is found that treatment can be discontinued as result of clinical improvement.

2. Have readily provoked angina on effort. Mild angina on effort has not been regarded as a reason for non-inclusion.

3. Have frequent ectopic complexes on the electrocardiograph (ECG) during or after exercise, unless these can be abolished by treatment.

4. Show little interest in the programme at the outset, or raise a lot of objections to taking part. Inability to 'find the time' is often a euphemism for lack of interest.

5. Have already made a good adjustment to their disorder and who, by the nature of their work, are already very physically active in their working hours.

INITIAL EVALUATION OF PATIENTS BY THE PHYSIOTHERAPIST

The first interview with the patient should be used to form an opinion about his probable level of physical fitness and general interests, as well as providing the opportunity for the physiotherapist to explain the purpose and content of the programme.

The following points should be inquired into:

1. *Current physical activity.* This not only indicates physical ability but may also define those patients who tend to be over-cautious (and perhaps over-anxious) or over-enthusiastic, allowing the physiotherapist to adapt the programme accordingly.

2. *Physical activity prior to the attack.* Information gained as a result of this question may be used in the rehabilitation of the patient. Thus the patient who previously played tennis or golf may be gradually able to resume his sport along with other aspects of the programme.

3. *Other interests.* Activities such as country dancing, deer-stalking and boating may have value in rehabilitation if the patient is keen to resume them.

4. *Occupation.* Obviously a sedentary worker will require a different programme to the manual worker. In addition, it may be useful to point out that the use of stairs in preference to a lift at the place of work may provide another source of exercise.

5. *Geography of the home.* In our experience this may make a lot of difference to the patient's efforts to increase mobility on returning from hospital. Thus early efforts at taking a walk may be inhibited if he lives half way up a steep hill or has to cope with flights of steps.

6. *Complications.* As will be mentioned later, modification of the programme may be necessary for those patients having other physical disabilities. It is wise

37

to elicit details of such conditions from the patient at first interview and thus avoid difficulties later. The two most likely to be encountered in coronary patients are degenerative joint disease and further signs of arterial disease, particularly intermittent claudication.

CLINICAL METHODS USED IN EVALUATION

In addition to a normal clinical examination, with particular attention to the cardiovascular and loco-motor systems, some sort of simple exercise test is necessary. This gives the team an objective impression of the patient's response to the stress of mild exercise and also allows monitoring of the ECG during and immediately after exercise. We have used an electrically-braked bicycle ergometer for this purpose (Elema-Schönander design), although mechanically-braked versions can also be used. A load of 500 kilopondmeters per minute (kpm/min) for three minutes at a pedalling speed of 60 revolutions per minute is tolerated by most patients who, on other grounds, appear likely to be suitable for the programme. Patients suspected of being particularly unfit may be started on a lower load of, say, 300 kpm/min. The test should not be done within two hours of a heavy meal. During the exercise the electro-cardiograph leads are kept in place and, with suitable equipment, recordings can be made while the patient is pedalling. The patient is asked to stop pedalling if he experiences any untoward symptoms such as shortness of breath, palpitations or more than slight angina and not to attempt to push himself beyond what he feels are his limits.

An alternative to a bicycle ergometer test is a stepping test, in which the patient steps on and off a platform of adjustable height. In spite of the cheapness of this equipment, the step test makes for difficulties in ECG monitoring during exercise, unless telemetering facilities are available. The Harvard step test is described in detail by De Vries (see Bibliography).

It is advisable for all initial tests to be done in the presence of, or within easy call of, the physician. A couch or bed should be handy in the room and the staff involved in the work should be familiar with the principles of emergency cardio-respiratory resuscitation. Defibrillation equipment should also be accessible and drugs for emergency use such as glyceryl trinitrate and pro-cainamide or lignocaine.

It is emphasised that the method of testing described here is not designed to measure physical fitness in terms such as PWC150 (physical work capacity at a heart rate of 150/min). Such determinations are more time-consuming and carry some increased risk to the patient but may be carried out by experienced investigators under carefully controlled conditions. The test we use as routine simply has a screening value, in that patients who show the unfavourable features mentioned above under a modest working load are not deemed suitable for the exercise programme, unless later testing shows some spontaneous improvement.

Electrocardiographic recordings should be made at intervals after the completion of exercise and it has been our practice to continue recording until the heart rate has returned to near resting levels. The value of this was once dramatically revealed when a patient developed a ventricular tachycardia six minutes after the end of a routine follow-up test, after having been in the pro-gramme for a year. Provision for filing the ECG records must be made, and it is helpful if untoward symptoms are noted on the ECG paper if they occur and also such details as the load used.

39

Once the suitability of a patient has been defined, the physician makes a point of explaining the purpose of the programme in simple terms to the patient. The possible benefits are outlined and a generally optimistic attitude taken. At the same time, no attempt is made to imply that participation in the programme is going to carry any guarantee of immunity from further heart attacks. We do suggest that the physically fit person is better placed to withstand a further attack should it occur. We also make a determined effort to make patients give up smoking and, where appropriate, reduce weight.

The exercise programme is two-phased. There is an initial scheme of formal exercises which increase joint mobility, strengthen muscle groups and gradually increase cardiovascular endurance; this part of the programme is described in detail in the next section. When a patient has worked his way through the formal programme, he is introduced to the idea of participation in swimming-pool activities and later such games as badminton and table-tennis. By introducing a 'fun' component into the programme a high degree of acceptability becomes possible and the weekly, or twice-weekly, gymnasium sessions are enjoyable occasions which many patients would be disappointed to miss. In addition they are encouraged to do their home programme as well. Some patients prefer to arrange their own activities and this they are encouraged to do, some playing golf regularly, some jogging or taking part in country dancing. These patients are followed up at intervals, since this helps to maintain motivation.

Patients are also reminded that they can help maintain their level of physical fitness by such measures as avoiding the use of the car where possible, always walking at a smart pace and avoiding the use of lifts.

CHAPTER 6

The Formal Exercise Programme

FORMAL EXERCISE is valuable in the early treatment of suitable convalescent coronary patients. Enthusiasm for this form of exercise is understandably fairly short-lived with many people and, if the idea of rehabilitation of a patient suffering from coronary heart disease is seen as a long-term one, the exercises may often have to be superseded by more general or sporting activities. It is helpful to find out where the patient's interests lie in this regard before starting him on a programme.

The formal exercises should not be too numerous or difficult, or lack obvious purpose, as even the most enthusiastic patient will tend to weary of them as time passes. The effects desired from a physical point of view should be able to be achieved with a fairly easy and quickly performed set of exercises using little or no equipment. The exercises should not be so complex that they are not easily remembered—or cannot be

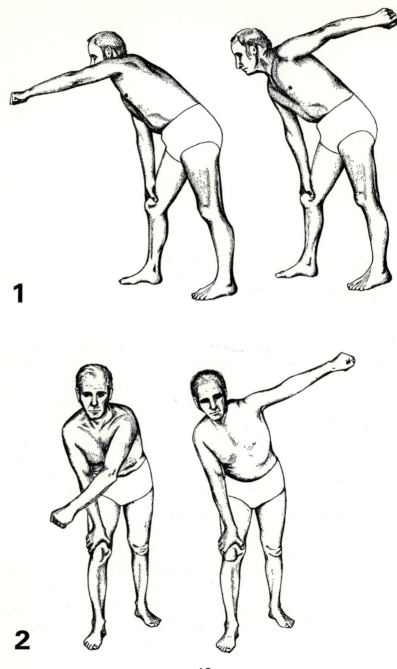

1

2

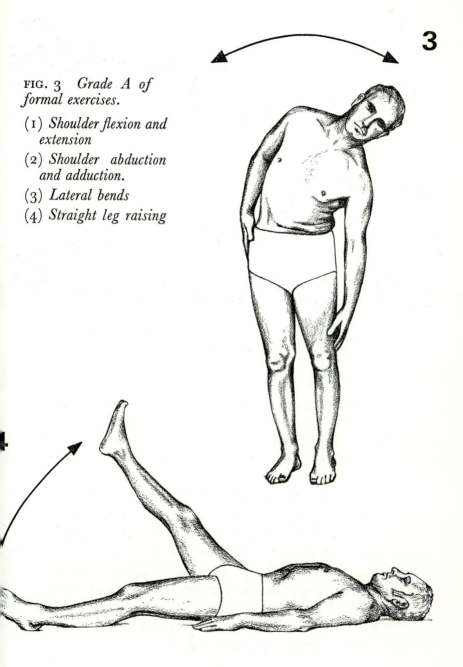

3

FIG. 3 *Grade A of formal exercises.*

(1) *Shoulder flexion and extension*
(2) *Shoulder abduction and adduction.*
(3) *Lateral bends*
(4) *Straight leg raising*

43

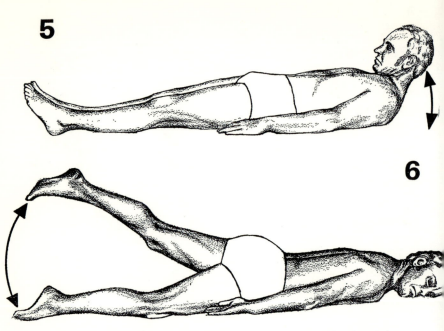

FIG. 3 *Grade A of formal exercises:* (5) *Head raising.* (6) *Prone lying; hip extension.*

performed in the limited confines of a small bathroom, an important factor in maintaining adherence.

The programme we have used has been developed over the past two years as the needs of the various patients became clear.

The exercise programme is divided into three grades, the contents of which are shown in Figures 3, 4 and 5. Those included in the first group, Grade A, are simply mobility exercises together with mild strengthening for the muscles of the trunk and legs. Stepping on to a stool provides a simple cardiovascular endurance exercise.

Grade B maintains mobility and introduces more strengthening exercises as well as a progression of the endurance exercise (running on the spot).

Grade C has fewer exercises requiring greater endurance, which are kept as the 'maintenance' list when a reasonable level of physical fitness has been achieved and the patient has been involved in other general activities.

We feel that it is important that shoulder mobility exercises and strengthening of the abdominal and quadriceps muscles be included in any programme for coronary heart disease patients, the former being aimed at reducing the likelihood of frozen shoulder in such patients and the latter aimed at improving these frequently weak muscles in middle-aged men.

While exercises are needed to strengthen spinal muscle groups, extreme flexion and extension manoeuvres are not advised because of the hazards of intervertebral disc damage in middle-aged patients. Thus back extension was excluded from the programme as it appeared to produce an exacerbation of symptoms attributable to spinal changes in some patients. In our opinion flexibility of approach is the keynote to success in the programme, so the exercises are readily modified to suit the individual. The three 'grades' provide a useful division but are not rigidly adhered to. Thus, following initial assessment, some of the younger patients may start on Grade B, plus mobility exercises from Grade A calculated to use all major joints and muscle groups; having achieved a degree of agility with these, they may progress to Grade C. Alternatively, a patient with a shoulder disability may retain exercises encouraging mobility of the joint throughout; and a patient with an osteo-arthritic knee or hip may have to exclude some of the stronger, weight-bearing exercises.

Progression in the number of times exercises are carried out also needs to be flexible. A suggestion is made as to the number of times each exercise should be

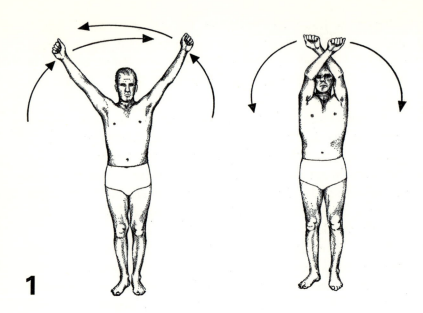

1

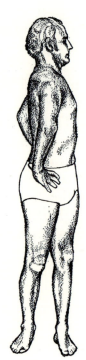

2

FIG. 4 *Grade B of formal exercises.*

(1) *Bilateral arm circumduction*

(2) *Hip twists*

(3) *Head and shoulder raising*

(4) *Side lying; hip abduction*

(5) *Press-ups from knees*

46

3

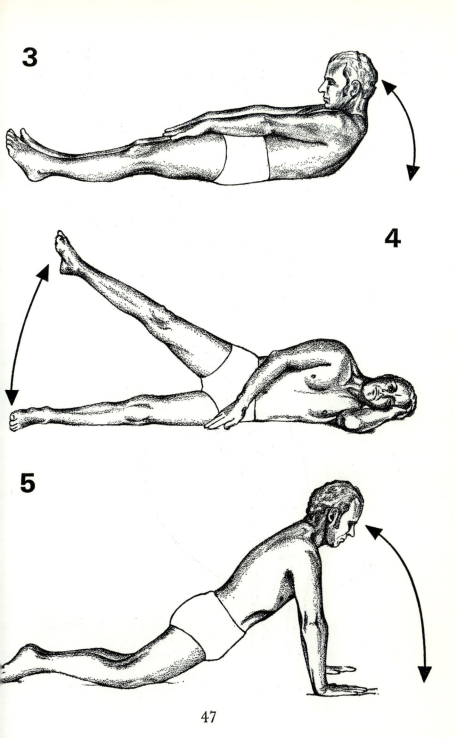

4

5

performed but the patient is told to extend himself to a point where he feels further exercise *may* produce symptoms; but he should avoid producing angina or excessive breathlessness. Patients appear to be very aware of their limitations and, having had the above clearly explained to them, will rarely overdo things. Occasionally the overcautious patient may not extend himself sufficiently and if, on discussion, progression appears slower than usual, it is wise to have the patient perform his list, checking the pulse rate before and after. We do not believe that a heart rate of 150 is necessary before improved cardiac performance will result;[3] this is an arbitrary figure and does not appear to allow for variations in resting levels. Obviously in a

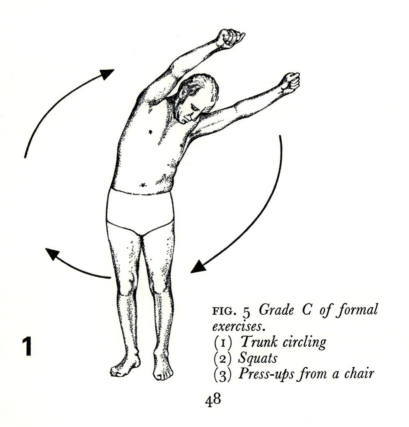

1

FIG. 5 *Grade C of formal exercises.*
(1) *Trunk circling*
(2) *Squats*
(3) *Press-ups from a chair*

48

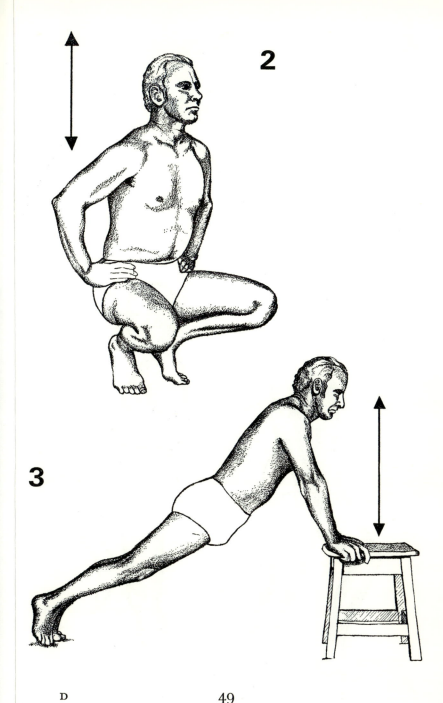

2

3

a time for these sessions which allows patients to attend after working hours (patients have frequently recommenced employment at the same time as starting the programme), but occasionally this is not possible and the patients can manage with only fortnightly or monthly visits. The weekly meetings allow for supervision, provide opportunities for the physician to watch closely the patient's reactions, as well as allowing the patients to participate in the exercises as a group.

Conditions involving the lower limbs demand ingenuity on the part of the physiotherapist in providing exercises that are predominantly non-weight-bearing and yet will still extend the cardiovascular system sufficiently to be of benefit. If the patient is able to participate regularly in swimming activities, this provides a partial substitute but may have the disadvantage of not being able to be performed quite so easily or so often.

Two other features which may cause alteration to the programme are the patient's age and sex. Although the majority of patients are men between the ages of forty and sixty-five, one is likely to encounter both younger and older men as well as a small percentage of women.

The patient under forty may sometimes be otherwise physically fit and perhaps still active in a sport. He may be able to be channelled back into this, perhaps in a modified capacity. Rugby and association football enthusiasts can still maintain a reasonable level of physical fitness by perhaps taking part in the sport as a coach. Patients in this age group appear to be more prone to anxiety because of their relative youth, and have more difficulty in adjusting to their condition; it is therefore important to gain their confidence and maintain their enthusiasm.

On the other hand, patients over the age of sixty-five may suffer from other physical disabilities with more general limitations to physical fitness but they must still be encouraged to do as much of the programme as is reasonably possible.

Women patients present a different problem. They tend to show greater reluctance to participate in callisthenics, especially when over the age of forty. They are not always able to be collected together for group activities as their free time is variable, depending on their family responsibilities. It is probably true to say that adherence is not likely to be as good as that of the men. Once again it is important to gain their confidence, but in our experience the physiotherapist may have to accept that a very little exercise is better than none at all. When numbers are sufficient, 'club' activities probably provide the best means of exercise for women.

It is important to remember that walking and the cardiovascular endurance exercise are essential parts of the formal programme. To ensure that the patient gets most benefit from these activities, a few suggestions can be made to improve their effectiveness. Walking should be done briskly; a leisurely stroll over even a considerable distance is not likely to produce such a good effect. It is helpful to the patient to suggest that he measure approximately a half or one mile and time himself walking this distance. Provided that it does not include a steep grade, an improvement in time should be aimed at. Obviously a limit will be reached and then distance may be increased. It goes without saying that the patient should never walk at a speed or over a distance that produces angina or excessive dyspnoea. Our best performers walk a mile in approximately twelve minutes, having begun at twenty minutes. With the endurance exercises, we suggest that the patient counts the number of steps taken or the amount of running on the spot he can do without provoking symptoms but nevertheless feeling that he has been extended. At later sessions he should try to improve on this number. The physiotherapist must make sure that the first stepping exercise is not done too slowly, otherwise the patient can do it indefinitely. When running on the spot is performed, it must be done thoroughly, i.e. knees well up, to get the maximum effect from the exercise.

In conclusion it must be pointed out that the formal exercise programme provides activity of a constant nature, involving all muscles and joints of the body. The aim is to increase gradually the daily physical activity and, having reached a reasonably high level, maintain it reguarly. Ultimately many activities may go to make up this regular exercise; in the initial stages a supervised formal exercise programme achieves this more than adequately.

THE SWIMMING POOL

It has been usual for us to introduce patients to activities in the swimming pool only when they are able to perform adequately the third grade of exercises, i.e each exercise approximately 20-25 times at a brisk pace, running-on-the-spot 100-150 times (both of these twice a day), and walking one to two miles daily, time and weather permitting.

There are a number of reasons for such caution. Firstly, because of the safety consideration; secondly, because close supervision of an individual in the pool is not always possible; thirdly, swimming is a complex activity putting considerable demands on the cardiovascular system.

Close supervision is maintained as far as possible in the first two or three sessions in the pool, the patient being given formal exercises to do which are an extension

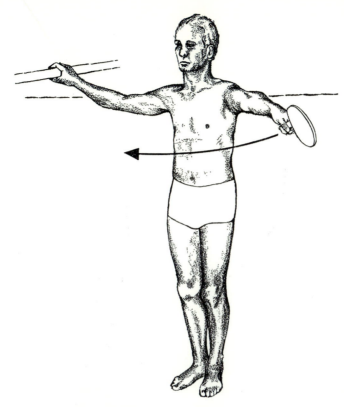

FIG. 6 *Pool exercises:* (1) *Horizontal abduction and adduction with bats.*

of those in the previous part of the programme. These are followed by a general activity in inflated rubber inner tubes with other patients. The patient is advised to stay in the water for no longer than half an hour and is dissuaded from taking part in competitive games as described elsewhere until both physician and patient are confident of his ability in the water.

The formal exercises we have used are shown in Figures 6 and 7. They include shoulder movements resisted by the use of hand-held bat; hip and knee

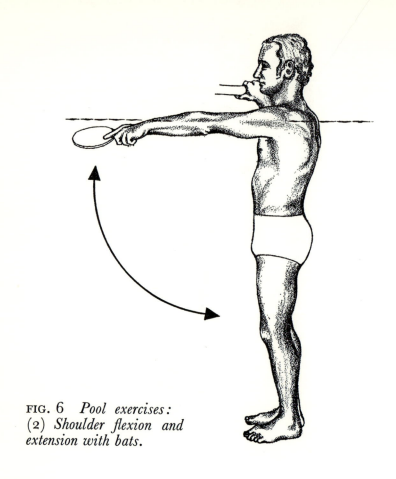

FIG. 6 *Pool exercises:*
(2) Shoulder flexion and
extension with bats.

movements resisted by floats on the feet; and trunk
flexion and extension resisted by floats. We have found
the inflated rubber tubes to be of the greatest assistance
with coronary patients. They allow mobility without
excessive effort; they encourage shoulder movements;
and they allow a non-swimmer to take part in the same
activities as a swimmer. One cautionary note is necessary, however. The supporting rubber tube encourages
relaxation and the physiotherapist must make sure that
real activity is maintained. One should also note that

56

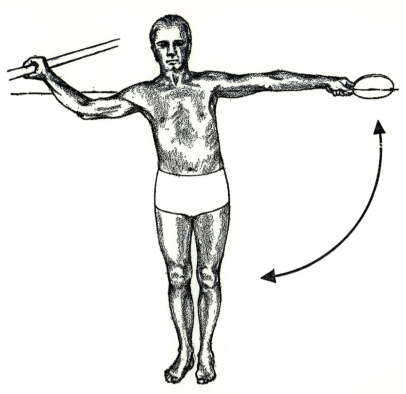

FIG. 6 *Pool exercises: (3) Shoulder abduction and adduction with bats.*

supervision of the patients must be carefully carried out, as in the excitement of group activities the supervisor may forget to keep a watchful eye on all involved.

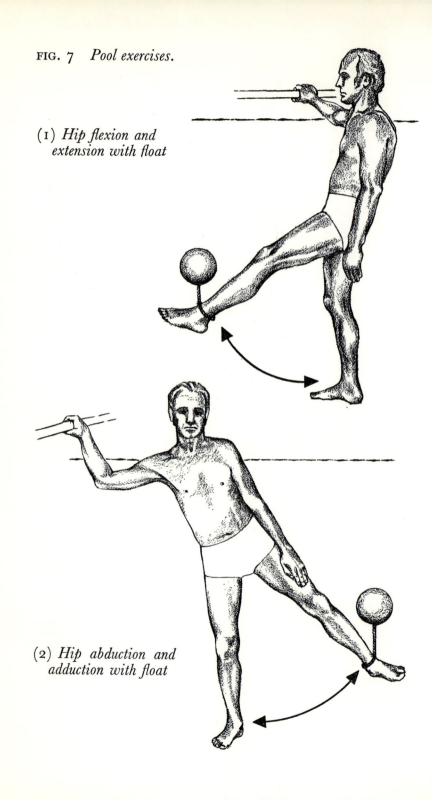

FIG. 7   *Pool exercises.*

(1) *Hip flexion and extension with float*

(2) *Hip abduction and adduction with float*

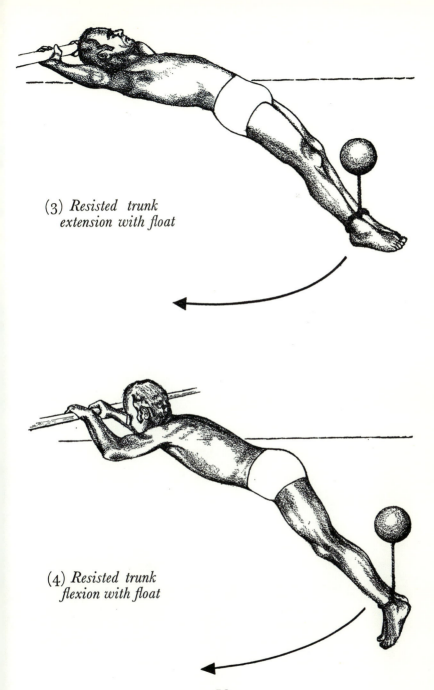

(3) *Resisted trunk extension with float*

(4) *Resisted trunk flexion with float*

59

CHAPTER 7

Epidemiological
Considerations

INFORMATION from various sources indicates clearly that coronary heart disease is the major cause of death in affluent communities. In the United Nations *Statistical Yearbook* 1967 it is recorded that the annual cardiovascular deaths per 100,000 males (aged 55-64 years) were 743 for the United Kingdom, 889 for New Zealand and 933 for the United States. The highest recorded figure was for Finland with 1037, the lowest for Jordan with 49 per 100,000. It is noted that in urbanised and industrial nations one-third of all deaths in the age group 45-64 are due to ischaemic heart disease.

It can be seen, therefore, that in the New Zealand community alone there are approximately 12,000 deaths annually from all forms of cardiovascular disease, compared with approximately 3600 deaths from all forms of cancer. In addition to the patients who succumb there are approximately four times as many who recover from coronary heart disease but suffer temporary or permanent disablement as a result. It is estimated by the New Zealand National Heart Foundation that heart disease probably costs the community approximately $100 m. per annum.

As ischaemic heart disease accounts for about one-third of all cardiovascular mortality, a reduction of a few per cent in its incidence would save the country millions of dollars annually, to say nothing of the saving in human suffering caused in families by illness or bereavement.

Clearly the main assault on coronary heart disease must lie in the field of prevention, and considerable research is being carried out in many countries to try to define the cause or causes of the disease. In relation to the possible causes so far studied there appears to be reasonable uniformity of opinion in regard to the harmful effects of cigarette smoking and of high blood pressure in provoking heart attacks.

The effect of dietary factors, such as a high intake of animal fat or of sugar, or both, is more controversial but on the evidence drawn both from epidemiological studies and from experimental work there are good grounds for believing that dietary factors play some part in causing the disease. It may be that the importance of the dietary factor differs in different communities.

Many workers in the field of cardiovascular disease consider that physical activity is of importance in reducing the incidence of the disease. The evidence for this view derives from epidemiological studies which show that, on the whole, workers who are physically active in their work have less coronary heart disease than colleagues in the same industry or public service who are relatively sedentary. However, it must be remembered that a good deal of self-selection is involved in choice of occupation. A man who chooses to be a postal delivery man rather than, say, a sorting clerk may be indirectly expressing a constitutional make-up which, of itself, is less coronary-prone.

In spite of the difficulties in interpreting epidemiological data, experimental evidence on man and animals has provided indirect grounds for thinking that physical exercise may help to prevent or delay either the development of coronary atherosclerosis or the event of myocardial infarction itself. The evidence rests on the findings, for instance, that physical exercise reduces the levels of some plasma lipids which are probably of considerable importance in formation of the atheromatous plaques in the arteries. Furthermore, exercise alters the clotting factors in the blood in various ways and it can be speculated that since the process of fibrinolysis (which tends to dissolve thrombi) is enhanced by physical activity a tendency to thrombus formation could be offset by regular stimulation of fibrinolytic mechanisms.

It may also be of importance that the fit and active members of the community are less prone to obesity, which, while of itself of doubtful causative significance for heart disease, does at least seem to reduce the chances of survival in overweight victims of the disease.

If, as seems probable but not proven, physical activity does play a part in preventing or delaying the appearance of coronary heart disease, then sooner or later the question will be posed, 'What type of exercise and how much will provide immunity from coronary heart disease?' The answer to this question is not known at present, nor is it likely that a clear-cut answer will be available for a number of years. Information on the amount and frequency of exercise that is necessary to produce measurable changes in certain physiological factors is known. Thus Siegel and others[4] found that thirty minutes of effective training weekly produced measurable effects in middle-aged men. Whether this amount of training is enough to influence the course of coronary artery disease is simply not known.

DOES TOO MUCH EXERCISE ADVERSELY AFFECT THE HEART?

Many people, including clinicians, are convinced that severe excrcise may sometimes cause a heart attack. While this is a difficult association to prove, many doctors have encountered patients whose myocardial infarctions came on during or immediately after severe physical effort. However, as pointed out by Hellerstein,[5] controlled, regular physical activity appears to carry negligible risk, and at the time of writing no patient in the Dunedin programme has had a myocardial infarction in the course of supervised exercise.

It seems probable, therefore, that it is only severe exercise in the untrained person who already has diseased coronary arteries that carries a risk.

There is negligible evidence that severe physical activity has a harmful effect in the young person with a normal heart and coronary arteries.

CHAPTER 8

The Coronary Club

THE BELIEF that a programme of physical activity has a place in the long-term management of coronary patients prompted us to find a formula that would be acceptable to patients over many years.

It is reasonably certain that only very few patients would maintain lasting interest in home callisthenics once the motivation provided by a recent coronary attack had worn off. Prolonged interest in some sort of physical programme would depend on their taking part in an activity that provided its own reward in the form of pleasant exercise carried out in the company of people in the same age group.

The foregoing considerations led to our proposing that the patients form themselves into a club. This club would be responsible for the maintenance of communication between patients regarding the activity programme, the provision of any extra equipment that patients might need, the collection of membership dues to provide extra amenities and the organisation of any other activities that patients might deem necessary.

In the Dunedin programme the club continued to use the gymnasiums and swimming pool available in the Department of Physiotherapy but provided its own equipment. It is quite conceivable that the club would have run just as well with rented or borrowed facilities provided in other ways.

ACTIVITIES

As indicated elsewhere, the chief activities to date of the Coronary Club have consisted of table tennis, badminton and a pool activity. The pool activity that has proved very popular consists of a kind of water polo in which the players are divided into two teams. Each player sits in an inflated inner tube and propels himself about the pool with his hands. Goal-posts can be made by a handyman in the group and placed about thirty feet apart in the shallow end of the pool. If there are more than three or four players per team, coloured skull caps, as worn by surf teams, will help players to distinguish team mates. The object of the game is to get the ball through the opposing team's goal. Rules can be made as simple or as elaborate as required. The referee in our programme is usually the physician, physiotherapist or a medical student. The great advantages of this game are that non-swimmers play on an equal footing with swimmers, the game enjoys considerable popularity and is sufficiently physically demanding, but nevertheless gives opportunities for patients to take things quietly on the sidelines if angina occurs. We have found that approximately 10-15 minutes play each way provides a good exercise spell. This game can be very energetic and we generally recommend some introductory pool exercises for newcomers (see pp. 55-7) as a preliminary to taking part in the game.

So far outdoor activities have not been a part of the Dunedin programme, although it is notable that some physicians in this field, Gottheiner for example,[6] have their patients taking part in strenuous outdoor games, sometimes of a highly competitive nature. It is probable that climatic factors will exert considerable influence on the range of activities suitable for inclusion in physical programmes for coronary patients and warmer areas may well be able to devise outdoor activities that would be unsuitable in Dunedin. The sport of orienteering, for example, would appear to be well suited to the physically active coronary patient but this suggestion was not popularly received by our patients. It is possible that it could be introduced by an enthusiastic physical educationist with experience of the sport in an area with fairly equable climate.

UNSUITABLE GAMES

There is at present an ill-defined feeling among physicians concerned with rehabilitation that some games are probably unsuitable for coronary patients although they may be ideal for maintaining physical fitness in normal persons. These consist mainly of sports where there is a considerable degree of person-to-person conflict such as occurs in judo, graeco-roman wrestling and fencing. Squash rackets is also probably unsuitable, except perhaps in selected patients who have been very good at the sport and were active at it before suffering an infarct. Even then they would probably be ill advised to play competitively again. Games that make insufficient demands on cardiovascular endurance may be unsuitable for a different reason. We would not regard bowls as suitable, nor, for that matter, golf when played in leisurely style on a flat course.

Ballroom dancing would probably be unsuitable on the whole, whereas Scottish country dancing and square dancing might well be ideal.

CHAPTER 9

The Physical and Psychological Effects of the Exercise Programme on Coronary Patients

As ALREADY INDICATED, there is currently no satisfactory scientific evidence that exercise programmes alter the risk of the development of further coronary attacks. This has not prevented medical scientists in this field from expressing optimistic but unsupported opinions on the probable value of such programmes.

Any doctor who contemplates mounting the sort of programme we have outlined, however, may well want reassurance that he is doing something more than merely running a pleasant but useless and time-consuming social club for his patients.

A number of studies have now been reported which indicate unequivocally that physical training produces measurable changes in haemodynamic, respiratory and metabolic parameters similar to those produced by comparable training in non-cardiac volunteers. [7] [8] [9] [10] [11] [12] The increase in working capacity that these studies record is complemented by the reported observation, which we can confirm in our own patients, that angina of effort is often less easily provoked, or may be lost altogether in trained patients.

The following data is drawn from a preliminary analysis of our own data and indicates the effect of as little as three months' training on our patients. Thus it was found that at a standard load the mean exercise heart rate in 22 patients dropped from 126 to 117 beats per minute, while the mean time for return of the heart rate to its resting level fell from 3·1 minutes to 2·4 minutes in the same group of patients. Both results were extremely unlikely to be due to chance by statistical analysis. Physical fitness can therefore be enhanced by regular training in coronary patients, as noted by others.

DOES EXERCISE REDUCE UNFAVOURABLE FEATURES?

Optimism in the value of physical fitness would be heightened if it could be shown that certain unfavourable characteristics frequently seen in coronary patients were improved by exercise. Some observations from the medical literature on the effect of physical training on patients are given below.

EFFECT ON BLOOD PRESSURE

Since high blood pressure affects the outcome in coronary heart disease it is of interest to note that a fall in blood pressure has been attributed to increased physical fitness by some authorities.[13] [14] [15] [16]

EFFECT ON SERUM LIPIDS

As indicated previously, high levels of some blood lipids are believed to play an important part in the development of the lesions of atherosclerosis. There is some suggestion that exercise does reduce some, if not all, plasma lipids, [17] [18] [19] [20] [21] [22] although in New Zealand a study of normal middle-aged males did not support the view.[23] It is possible that dietary changes produced by exercise might make for difficulties in interpretation of the data.

EFFECT ON OBESITY

Physical exercise has at best only marginal value in the control of obesity. While athletic individuals are seldom obese (with the notable exception of Japanese wrestlers), physical activity without the use of dietary measures is not a very good way to lose weight. In a New Zealand study of middle-aged males a jogging programme which was associated with marked changes in physical fitness was only accompanied by a mean weight loss of $1 \cdot 7$ lb in 32 men over 5 months' training.[23] There was a $13 \cdot 8$ per cent reduction in skinfold thickness (a measure of subcutaneous fat). It could be speculated that some of the apparent failure to lose weight was due to an increase in muscle bulk as the result of training.

From the foregoing observations it seems difficult to draw the conclusion that physical activity offers anything more than slight changes in improving those factors known to be associated with increased risk of the development of coronary heart disease. However, it may well be that beneficial effects occur in other and less easily measured ways, such as by effects on blood coagulability. In any event it would seem improbable that any exercise programme would alter the arterial changes that are seen in affected patients. What may happen, however, is that the circumstances that bring about the definitive event of myocardial infarction or onset of serious rhythm disturbance may be less easily provoked in the trained patient.

PSYCHOLOGICAL EFFECTS

As noted by Hellerstein[16] and by Wynn,[24] many coronary patients have emotional problems, such as anxiety and depression as a result of their illness.

It is not difficult to see why this should be so. The heart looms so large in emotive language that such expressions as 'dying of a broken heart' assume a real and sinister significance to the coronary patient. The patient's friends and relations may, by their various attitudes, encourage the patient in his fears that he may not have long to live or be liable to die suddenly. The over-solicitous and anxious spouse or friend may transfer some of this anxiety to the patient; he may come to accept that he is an invalid in need of continual and watchful care and subscribe to the irrational notion that he will die if he so much as raises his arms above his head.

As pointed out by Wynn, much needless anxiety can probably be avoided by early and, if necessary, repeated discussion between the patient and his doctor about the nature of the disease. The acquisition of wild and frightening misconceptions may thus be avoided. This explanation should be regarded as the first step in rehabilitation.

Part of the patient's anxiety undoubtedly rests in uncertainty about his or her physical capacity. Will he be able to do his normal job again or, in the case of a woman, be able to cope with the children and the housework? The patient may be hesitant to test his physical limits and may tend, therefore, to move and work at a restricted pace, not only below his untrained capacity but well below what he might achieve with the aid of physical re-education. Thus for many coronary patients the realisation that with physical training their capacity may be well up to all the normal demands of their working and leisure activities comes as something of a revelation. The participation in group activities in which they can share a sense of identity with other patients who have faced and overcome the same emotional difficulties also appears to have a strong beneficial effect on mood. Hellerstein[16] recorded a significant reduction in depression in trained patients as measured by special psychological testing. This agrees with our own subjective impression of increased optimism and sense of well being in our patients.

At this point it must be stated that while it is probable that any psychological effect of the programme may be due to the physical training itself, we cannot discount the perhaps considerable effect of other factors. Thus the interest of an enthusiastic medical team, the camaraderie of the training group, the feeling of making some positive contribution to one's own health may of themselves have potent effects on mood and optimism quite independently of the effect of the physical programme. We take the view that the academic considerations on this issue are perhaps less important than the undoubtedly beneficial effects on the patients. Doubtless the question will ultimately be resolved by careful studies in which the contribution of the non-physical aspects of the programme will be defined.

Most physicians, physiotherapists and medical students who have seen the patients at their activities are impressed, and sometimes surprised, at the vigour with which many patients are able to perform. It seems inescapable that the attitude of patients to their disease would often reflect that of their physician. Doctors who are familiar with this type of therapy would be liable to transmit a much more optimistic attitude to coronary patients under their care.

Bibliography

1. Currens, J. H. and White, P. D. (1961), *New England J. Med.*, 265, 988.
2. Eckstein, R. W. (1957), *Circulation Research*, 5, 230.
3. Åstrand, P-O. (1967), *Canad. Med. Ass. J.*, 96, 907.
4. Siegel, W., Blomqvist, A. and Mitchell, J. H. (1970), *Circulation*, 41, 19.
5. Hellerstein, H. K. (1969), *Circulation* (Supp. 4), 40, IV, 124.
6. Gottheiner, V. (1966), in *Prevention of Ischaemic Heart Disease* (Charles C. Thomas, Illinois).
7. Hellerstein, H. K., Burlando, B., Hirsch, E. Z., Plotkin, F. H., Feil, G. H., Winkler, O., Marik, S. and Margolis, N. (1965), *Circulation* (Supp. 2), 32, 110.
8. Varnauskas, E., Bergman, H., Houk, P. and Björntorp, P. (1966), *Lancet*, 2, 8.
9. Frick, M. H. and Katila, M. (1968), *Circulation*, 37, 192.
10. Clausen, J. P., Larsen, O. A. and Trap-Jensen, J. (1969), *Circulation*, 40, 143.
11. Sloman, G., Pitt, A., Hirsch, E. Z. and Donaldson, A. (1965), *Med. J. Aust.*, 1, 4.

12. Bergman, H., Björntorp, P., Houk, P., Varnauskas, E. and Westerlund, A. (1966), *Läkartidningen*, 63, 407.

13. Naughton, J., Shanbour, K., Armstrong, R., McCoy, J. and Lategola, M. T. (1966), *Arch. Int. Med.*, 117, 541.

14. Berkson, D., Whipple, I., Sime, D., Lerner, H., Bernstein, I., MacIntyre, W. and Stamler, J. (1967), *Circulation*, 36, 67.

15. Mann, G. V., Garrett, H., Billings, F., Murray, H. and Fahri, A. (1967), *Circulation* (Supp. 2), 36, 181.

16. Hellerstein, H. K. (1968), *Bull. N.Y. Acad. Sci.*, 44, 1028.

17. Montoye, H. J., Van Huss, W. D., Brewer, W. D., Jones, E. M., Ohlson, M. A., Mahoney, E. and Olsen, H. (1959), *Am. J. Clin. Nutr.*, 7, 139.

18. Holloszy, J. O., Skinner, J. S., Toro, G. and Cureton, T. K. (1964), *Am. J. Cardiol.*, 14, 753.

19. Carlson, L. A., and Mossfeldt, F. (1964), *Acta. Physiol. Scand.*, 62, 51.

20. Shane, S. R. (1966), *Am. J. Cardiol.*, 18, 540.

21. Campbell, D. E. (1965), *J. Lipid Res.*, 6, 478.

22. Naughton, J. and McCoy, J. F. (1966), *J. Chron. Dis.*, 19, 727.

23. Hunter, J. D., Nye, E. R., O'Donnell, T. V. and Heslop, J. (1968), *New Zealand Med. J.*, 67, 288.

24. Wynn, A. (1967), *Med. J. Australia*, 2, 847.

Further useful sources of information are:

PHYSIOLOGY

De Vries, H. A. (1967), *Physiology of Exercise* (Staples, London).

Åstrand, P-O. and Rodahl, K. (1970), *Textbook of Work Physiology* (McGraw-Hill).

THERAPEUTIC ASPECTS OF EXERCISE

Karvonen, M. J. and Barry, A. J. (1967), *Physical Activity and the Heart*, (Charles C. Thomas, Illinois).

Raab, W. (1966), *Prevention of Ischaemic Heart Disease* (Charles C. Thomas, Illinois).

Appendix

SUGGESTED PROTOCOL FOR EXERCISE TESTING OF A POPULATION GROUP*
OPERATIONAL REQUIREMENTS

1. *Staff*

Exercise testing is a highly specialised task and must be performed by well trained personnel. The measurement of physiological parameters during exercise and the general conduct of work experiments should be learnt in an established laboratory of exercise physiology.

The doctor should select the proper loading pattern, watch the subjects for signs and symptoms indicating that exercise should be interrupted (see below under Safety Precautions, Sections 4 and 5) and interpret the ECG and other results, while the technicians and nurse should take care of the various analytical procedures and calculations, prepare the electrodes for ECG, take the anthropometric measurements, etc. However, if a

---

*Prepared by the Cardiovascular Diseases Unit, WHO, with the assistance of Professor K. Lange Andersen, Oslo, Professor H. Denolin, Brussels, and Dr E. Varnauskas, Göteborg.

79

simple exercise test is used involving stepping or pedalling a bicycle ergometer, with recording of the pulse rate, the ECG wave-form and perhaps the systemic blood pressure, but with no respiratory measurement, then one experienced person can take care of the whole procedure and may be able to test up to fifteen subjects a day.

2. *Equipment*

Ergometer (preferably a bicycle), electrocardiograph, sphygmomanometer, stop-watches, defibrillator and drugs (as a safety precaution), cardio-tachometer (optional), metronome (optional).

All instruments (bicycle ergometers, electrocardiographs, etc.) require careful and frequent calibration. Access to a proper workshop or other facilities for necessary servicing is therefore important. The repeatability and validity of proposed measurements (see Rose and Blackburn, *Cardiovascular Survey Methods*, WHO, 1968, for details) should be established by each team before a population survey is conducted.

3. *Types of Ergometers*

The steps or the mechanically-braked bicycle ergometer are the preferred instruments for population studies. Both the step test and the mechanical bicycle ergometer test fulfil most of the requirements of transportation, maintenance, calibration, task familiarity, relatively low cost, and subject's optimal performance. The steps, obviously, are the cheapest device. They can be constructed in any carpenter's workshop and present no transportation, calibration or maintenance problems. This test, however, may present some difficulty in the assessment of the mechanical efficiency of effort and, because of the broad movements of the subject, in the monitoring of ECG, blood pressure, heart rate, etc. It also requires a greater degree of co-operation and, perhaps, of neuromuscular co-ordination on the part of the subject. Also, it does not yield meaningful results unless accompanied by respiratory measurements. For the purpose of this trial the mechanically-braked bicycle ergometer is recommended.

In the usual type a frictional force is developed on or within the driving wheel, and the work performed is proportional to the product of the applied force and the total number of wheel revolutions. The source of friction is normally a weighted leather belt applied to the outer surface of the driving wheel, but models using weighted brake shoes have also been devised. In the simplest forms of machine the frictional force is either calculated from the difference between the applied weights and the reading of a spring balance, or is indicated by the position of a calibrated and weighted lever. More sophisticated machines permit the direct application of the desired load. Several problems may arise in the use of the simpler machines:

(a) The belt becomes hot, altering the co-efficient of friction, thus possibly giving rise to systematic errors.
(b) The system of belt, weights and levers forms a compound pendulum, and the spring balance or load indicator fluctuates wildly during vigorous effort.
(c) Inexperienced subjects may find difficulty in maintaining a constant rhythm.

Several types of bicycle ergometers are commercially available. One of the most popular simple designs is that of von Döbeln, in which the calibration is arranged so that a scale and pointer indicate the approximate work (in kilopondmeters, kpm) performed by one rotation of the ergometer wheel. The bicycle is connected to a rpm counter which records the number of ergometer wheel rotations during the test period, thus permitting estimation of the total work output during this period.

The bicycle should be so constructed as to allow the work rate (work performed per unit of time in kpm/min. or in watts) to be recorded, and to permit changes in the work rate while keeping the pedalling rate constant. It should have also a large rate indicator from which the patient can gauge his rate of pedalling, although some adults prefer to keep time with a metronome.

The pedal crank length should be 15-20 cm (for adults) and the height of the bicycle seat should be rapidly adjustable. The shape of the seat deserves attention—most people prefer a narrow seat.

WORK OUTPUT AND WORK RATE

Work output is usually expressed in kilopondmeters (kpm) or in kilogrammeters (kgm), which are equivalent in unit gravitation field. Work rate is expressed in kpm/min., kgm/min., or watts.

The conversion of kpm/min. into watts, or vice versa, can be made according to the equation: 1 watt = 6 kpm/min. (approx.), or 1 kpm/min. = 0·167 watts. Bicycle ergometers are usually factory-calibrated in any of these units. Detailed calibration instructions are supplied with the machine.

The total work output (W_t) during the whole testing period t can be calculated as follows:

$$W_t = w.a,$$

w being the work (indicated on the machine scale) performed during one rotation of the ergometer wheel and a the number of rotations of the wheel in time t (indicated by the rpm counter).

The work rate in kpm/min. would therefore be: W_t/t.

EXAMPLE OF PROTOCOL FOR CALCULATING WORK
RATE ON MECHANICAL BICYCLE ERGOMETER

Load on ergometer wheel, w			
Duration of exercise period, in minutes, t			
Number (a) of ergometer wheel rotations in time t			
Work rate in kpm/min.			

SAFETY PRECAUTIONS

Exercise tests are widely used and safe procedures, particularly when they are only performed to submaximal levels of effort. Nevertheless the possibility of accidents cannot be ruled out and some safety precautions should be taken into consideration.

A systematic investigation concerning the occurrence of complications in connection with exercise tests is not available. Occasional reports and personal communications disclose, however, that minor complications are not rare and that serious cardiovascular accidents, in a few instances fatal, have been observed. Vaso-vagal reactions seem to be quite frequent but, if injury is avoided, are usually benign, while cardiac arrhythmias, especially those of ventricular origin, are relatively rare but much feared. Acute cardiac failure is a rare complication observed in severely ill patients with chronic valvular heart disease, but sometimes also in healthy

83

subjects. Angina pectoris is usually accepted as a limit for workload increase and is not regarded as a complication except in status anginosus; if the electrocardiogram is monitored throughout the test, angina is rare in random population samples.

Experience suggests that the fatal outcome of the few known accidents is due to poor organisation of safety measures in connection with exercise testing in general. Since the occurrence of ventricular tachycardia or ventricular fibrillation is possible in apparently normal people, it is advisable that any team testing normal subjects should be well prepared for emergency situations and that appropriate emergency equipment be available.

1. *Personnel*

Although exercises at low work loads can in general be conducted by a single supervisor, the team responsible for testing should include at least two or three people, and a physician must be near at hand if none of these people is a physician. In this way accidents due to exhaustion may be prevented and possible emergency situations may be dealt with.

The members of the testing team must have a basic understanding of exercise physiology. They must be well acquainted with the testing procedure and the risks involved in different methods of testing. They must be able to recognise signs and symptoms of impending difficulties and be competent to initiate appropriate therapy without delay. Each member should be trained to recognise basic ECG abnormalities.

2. *Medical Facilities*

Each room must be equipped with a couch where the patient may lie. A defibrillator is one of the most important pieces of safety equipment, but probably it is not mandatory when testing a population group free from cardiovascular diseases, particularly if the strenuous, maximal tests are avoided. Emergency medicines must include drugs against arrhythmias (lidocain or procainamide and quinidine); against severe hypotension or shock (a pressor amine); against angina pectoris (nitroglycerin); and against acute cardiac failure (digitalis). Glucose/saline infusion sets should be available.

3. Medical Examination of the Patient

Prior to exercise a thorough medical history should be recorded. Physical examination should include the cardio-respiratory system, with competent evaluation of a classical 12-lead ECG recording (see below under 'Performance of Exercise Test', Section 3—page 91).

Continuous recording during exercise considerably increases both the safety of the test—by making it possible to stop it as soon as any significant electrical anomaly appears—and its validity—by revealing changes in the electrocardiogram which appear only at the commencement of the test or disappear rapidly after the end of the exercise. A continuation of recording for at least six minutes after exercise is desirable to detect anomalies which may appear only at a late stage or become accentuated during the post-exercise period.

4. Contra-indications to Exercise Testing

The test cannot be performed routinely if significant locomotor disturbances are present, since impaired neuromuscular function or skeletal abnormality may alter the subject's response to exercise.

Anxiety may decisively influence the circulatory

response to exercise and may also increase the heart's vulnerability to arrhythmias.

Manifest cardiac failure, symptoms and electrocardiographic signs of impending or acute myocardial infarction and myocarditis, and aortic stenosis are all contra-indications for exercise testing. Three months must elapse between an acute episode of myocardial infarction and exercise testing.

Acute infectious diseases, unstable metabolic conditions and the probability of recent pulmonary embolism are also considered as contra-indications to exercise testing.

Special precautions must be exercised when patients with the following conditions are being tested: arterial fibrillation or flutter, high degrees of atrio-ventricular block, left bundle branch block syndrome, and the Wolff-Parkinson-White syndrome.

5. *Indications for Stopping Exercise*

The discontinuation of the exercise should be considered immediately when (i) the subject starts complaining of increasing pain in the chest, severe dyspnoea, severe fatigue, faintness and claudication, (ii) when the subject shows clinical signs suggestive of an impending emergency situation, including pallor, cold moist skin, cyanosis, staggering, confusion in response to inquiries, the facies of cerebrovascular insufficiency and head-nodding. Each subject should be able to discontinue the test at his will, so as to minimise the danger of exhaustion, falls and cardio-circulatory accidents.

The exact limit of increase of systolic blood pressure as a result of exercise is unknown. An exaggerated increase (e.g. 230-250 mmHg, although readings up to 300 mmHg have been recorded without any hazard to the subject) in relation to age and to clinical conditions calls for stopping of the exercise test. Similarly, exertional hypotension or lack of the normal pressure increase during exercise constitutes a contra-indication to continued effort.

The ECG should be watched throughout the whole period of exercise test and, if facilities are available, an electronic signal average device is most helpful. The exercise test should be discontinued if the following ECG changes occur: paroxysmal suproventricular and ventricular arrhythmias, ventricular premature beats appearing before the end of the T-wave, conduction disturbances other than a slight AV-block, and ST-depression of horizontal or descending types greater than 0·1 mV. Arrhythmias frequently become more marked immediately on stopping exercise, and if in doubt, the investigator should always halt the test. Regardless of the heart rate that is expected to be attained, it is recommended to stop the exercise if the heart rate reaches the following values:

AGE	UPPER LIMITS	
20-29 years	170 beats/min.	
30-39 years	160	,, ,,
40-49 years	150	,, ,,
50-59 years	140	,, ,,
60 years and over	130	,, ,,

6. *Post-exercise Recovery Period*

The frequency of both minor and major complications, including arrhythmias, is probably greater during the recovery period than during the exercise itself. Postural hypotension may develop immediately after exercise which can also provoke arrhythmias. Rapid cooling of the body may further increase the heart's susceptibility to arrhythmias. Unless it is specifically necessary to make recovery observations, the exercise should be gradually tapered off and subjects should be seated in a semi-reclining chair to minimise postural problems. Neither cold nor hot showers should be allowed immediately after the completion of exercise. ECG should be monitored for at least five minutes.

ENVIRONMENTAL CONDITIONS

1. *Time of Day*

Many of the functions commonly measured during exercise tests, such as pulse rate and body temperature, show a pronounced circadian rhythm. During waking hours, a variety of factors also tend to have a harmful effect on human performance. High doses of tobacco, for instance, may lead to bronchospasm, tachycardia, and reduced peripheral blood flow; in certain specific occupational groups the tendency to bronchospasm is further enhanced by dusts encountered at work. Many subjects spend their working day standing, and this can lead to peripheral pooling of fluid, with an increase of extracellular water and a reduction of the central blood volume. For all these reasons, the time of day when the measurements are made is of some importance. Unfortunately, this factor is often determined by hours of employment, and is thus outside the control of the physician. Nevertheless the time of examination should always be recorded and, whether comparing an individual with himself or with another, every effort should be made to carry out the tests at a comparable time of the day.

2. *Environmental Temperature*

The critical range of environmental temperature is from 20° to 30°c; at 20°c almost all of the cutaneous

88

vessels are fully constricted, and at 30°C almost all are fully dilated. The influence of environmental temperature becomes less as the intensity of exercise is increased, since the exercise itself tends to demand full dilation of the cutaneous vessels. The heat load imposed by a given air temperature depends also upon the radiant heat load, the relative humidity, the air speed and the nature of the clothing worn during the test. If radiant heating is avoided and if the relative humidity is less than 60 per cent and the air is still, then the laboratory temperature should be kept in the range of 18° to 22°C (64 to 72°F). The upper limit can be increased by about 2°C if the effective temperature is reduced by use of a large fan.

Exercise tests are not normally conducted in a cold environment and should not be carried out if the room temperature is below 10°C.

3. *Clothing*

The deep body temperature can rise as much as 1°C during a 12-minute or 18-minute continuous sub-maximum test exercise. The free loss of heat from the body is thus important if unduly high pulse rates are not to be recorded during the final minutes of exercise. The maximum skin surface should thus be exposed, using light shorts where possible.

The subjects should wear their normal shoes, provided they are comfortable and suitable for pedalling. When exercise is performed barefoot or in gym shoes with low heels and poor ankle support, the chances of a sprained ankle or an injury of the Achilles tendon are substantially increased.

PERFORMANCE OF EXERCISE TEST

1. *Exercise*

For this type of population survey, it is suggested to use a submaximal test with increasing, multi-level work loads. It would be advisable to perform such tests more than once: the first time to familiarise the subject with the equipment and with the procedure, and a few more times afterwards in close daily succession so as to obtain mean values. This should be done both before and after the treatment.

The basic feature of an exercise test is that heart rate increases in linear relation to the increase both in work load and in oxygen uptake. The test is performed by having the subject exercising at three or four sub-maximal work loads and by recording the corresponding heart rates. Maximal work load will then be graphically extrapolated to maximal heart rate as described in detail below. For the sake of simplicity, no respiratory measurements will be taken, and oxygen uptake values will also be obtained by extrapolation. At maximal heart rate a fit subject is expected to yield a higher work output, and oxygen uptake, than an unfit one.

2. *Mode of Performance*

(a) After a pre-exercise medical examination, the subjects warm up for a few minutes by pedalling the bicycle at a low work load, e.g. 60 kpm/min.

(b) The height of the saddle pillar should be adjusted to the height of the subject so that the legs are almost fully stretched at the knee point when the ball of the foot is applied to the pedals and one pedal is at its lowest position. The subject should always remain seated and is not allowed to lift his body.

(c) The pedalling rate should be between 50 and 60 strokes/min., since this is the most comfortable rate for people of average fitness. This rate should be maintained, with the aid of the metronome or a tachometer, throughout the whole exercise period. The exercise proper then begins by setting the work load at fixed values as follows:

Adult men: 300 kpm/min.
600 ,, ,,
900 ,, ,,

For weak persons a better loading may be:
300 ,, ,,
450 ,, ,,
600 ,, ,,

(d) Three of such submaxial work loads should be performed, each lasting six minutes. A small pause may be allowed between the runs.

(e) The number of rotations on the ergometer wheel or on the pedal should be recorded for each of the six minute periods, and used in the calculations of work rate (see page 82).

3. *Monitoring of ECG and Heart Rate*

It is of advantage to record ECG during exercise; however, this procedure is left to the decision of the supervising investigator and is not considered mandatory. If ECG is recorded during exercise, it is not necessary to use a 12-lead system. A bipolar lead system is recommended, one (exploring) electrode in the V_5 position, the other (reference) fastened at the lower edge of the right scapula. The neutral electrode may be at the right arm. The selector switch at the ECG machine is set at lead 1. The reference electrode may also be placed at the symmetrical point on the right hemi-thorax (C5-C5R) or on the manubrium sterni (CM5). Correct preparation of the skin, by rubbing with ether and using special paste, is necessary.

Heart rate and ECG pattern are recorded during the last minute of each exercise period, although it may be advisable, as a safety procedure, to monitor these functions throughout the whole exercise period.

ECG wave pattern should be examined and coded according to the modified Minnesota code. When only heart rate is recorded, the paper speed may be set to 25 mm/sec. The heart rate may be conveniently found by measuring the distance between 7 R-waves (6 intervals) and applying the following formula:

$$\text{Heart rate} = \frac{a}{b} \times 60,$$

where a (in cm) is the distance between 7 beats and b is the paper speed in mm/min.

When ECG pattern is to be examined, a paper speed of 50 mm/sec. is recommended. In order to obtain a good record it may sometimes be useful to take the ECG immediately after cessation of exercise, and further to ask the subject to hold his breath for a few seconds of recording.

As to blood pressure, in most circumstances the only practical method of measurement is the cuff method. However, this has certain disadvantages when used during exercise, and only the systolic pressure can be assessed reasonably well.

4. *Evaluation of Results*

For the purpose of this trial one need only record the ECG. However, all signs and symptoms, as well as the laboratory findings that are relevant, should be recorded and evaluated.

As to the ECG findings, only an ST depression of more than 0·1 mV. and of 0·06 seconds duration beyond the J point (whether upsloping, horizontal, or down-sloping) can be considered as a sure sign of ECG abnormality.

5. *Termination of Exercise Test*

As mentioned under 'Safety Precautions' Section 6, the exercise should be tapered off rather than suddenly stopped, and the subject should be checked for possible electrocardiographic or other adverse reactions.

Immediately after termination of exercise the leads V_2, V_4 and V_5, I, II and III should be recorded in that order. The same recording should be done five minutes later and, if the heart rate has not yet decreased to below 100, again ten minutes after cessation of test.

NOTES

NOTES

NOTES